Carnivore Keto for Beginners (Poultry and Dessert Edition)

The best keto recipes for beginners

© Copyright 2021 - All rights reserved.

The content contained within this book may not be reproduced, duplicated or transmitted without direct written permission from the author or the publisher.

Under no circumstances will any blame or legal responsibility be held against the publisher, or author, for any damages, reparation, or monetary loss due to the information contained within this book. Either directly or indirectly.

Legal Notice:

This book is copyright protected. This book is only for personal use. You cannot amend, distribute, sell, use, quote or paraphrase any part, or the content within this book, without the consent of the author or publisher.

Disclaimer Notice:

Please note the information contained within this document is for educational and entertainment purposes only. All effort has been executed to present accurate, up to date, and reliable, complete information. No warranties of any kind are declared or implied. Readers acknowledge that the author is not engaging in the rendering of legal, financial, medical or professional advice. The content within this book has been derived from various sources. Please consult a licensed professional before attempting any techniques outlined in this book.

By reading this document, the reader agrees that under no circumstances is the author responsible for any losses, direct or indirect, which are incurred as a result of the use of information contained within this document, including, but not limited to, — errors, omissions, or inaccuracies.

Sommario

INTRODUCTION 8
POULTRY RECIPES 10
FESTIVE TURKEY ROULADEN 10
PAN-FRIED CHORIZO SAUSAGE 12
CHINESE BOK CHOY AND TURKEY SOUP 14
HERBY CHICKEN MEATLOAF 16
LOVELY PULLED CHICKEN EGG BITES 18
CREAMY MUSTARD CHICKEN WITH SHIRATAKI 20
PARSNIP & BACON CHICKEN BAKE 22
CHICKEN BAKE WITH ONION & PARSNIP 24
CUCUMBER-TURKEY CANAPES 26
BAKED CHICKEN SKEWERS WITH RUTABAGA FRIES 28
LOUISIANA CHICKEN FETTUCCINE 30
CHICKEN WRAPS IN BACON WITH SPINACH 33
373.   CAULI RICE & CHICKEN COLLARD WRAPS 35
374.   STUFFED PEPPERS WITH CHICKEN & BROCCOLI 37
GRILLED CHICKEN KEBABS WITH CURRY & YOGURT 39
CHICKEN WITH TOMATO AND ZUCCHINI 41
CREAM CHEESE & TURKEY PASTRAMI ROLLS 43
ALMOND CRUSTED CHICKEN ZUCCHINI STACKS 44
PALEO COCONUT FLOUR CHICKEN NUGGETS 46
CHICKEN FAJITA BOWLS 48
PROSCIUTTO-WRAPPED CHICKEN 50
CREAMY CHICKEN CORDON BLEU 52
CHEESY CHICKEN DRUMSTICKS 55
JAMAICAN CURRY CHICKEN DRUMSTICKS 58

PARMESAN DRUMSTICKS 60

CHICKEN LEGS WITH MAYO SAUCE 63

CHICKEN WITH CHEESE MUSHROOM SAUCE 66

CHICKEN CACCIATORE 69

SALSA CHICKEN LEGS 71

DESSERT RECIPES **73**

PEANUT BUTTER CHOCOLATE CAKE 73

CROCKPOT APPLE PUDDING CAKE 75

BROWNIE COOKIES 77

CHOCOLATE CARAMEL MONKEY BREAD 79

COFFEE CAKE 81

SLOW-COOKING APPLE PEAR CRISP 84

PERFECT CHEESECAKE 87

SLOW COOKING LEMON PASTRY 90

KEY LIME DUMP CAKE 93

CROCKPOT CANDY SAUCE 95

CHERRY PASTRY CROCKPOT 97

CROCKPOT PUMPKIN CAKE 99

BLUEBERRY CAKE 101

CROCKPOT STRAWBERRY DUMP CAKE 103

RED VELVET PIE 105

LEMON MOUSSE WITH LIME CREAM AND ROASTED NUTS 107

ALMOND PANNA COTTA 110

ALMOND WITH CHOCOLATE SAUCE AND CHERRY GARNISH 112

CUISINE BROWNIES 115

CAKE CRUST 117

CONCLUSION..**119**

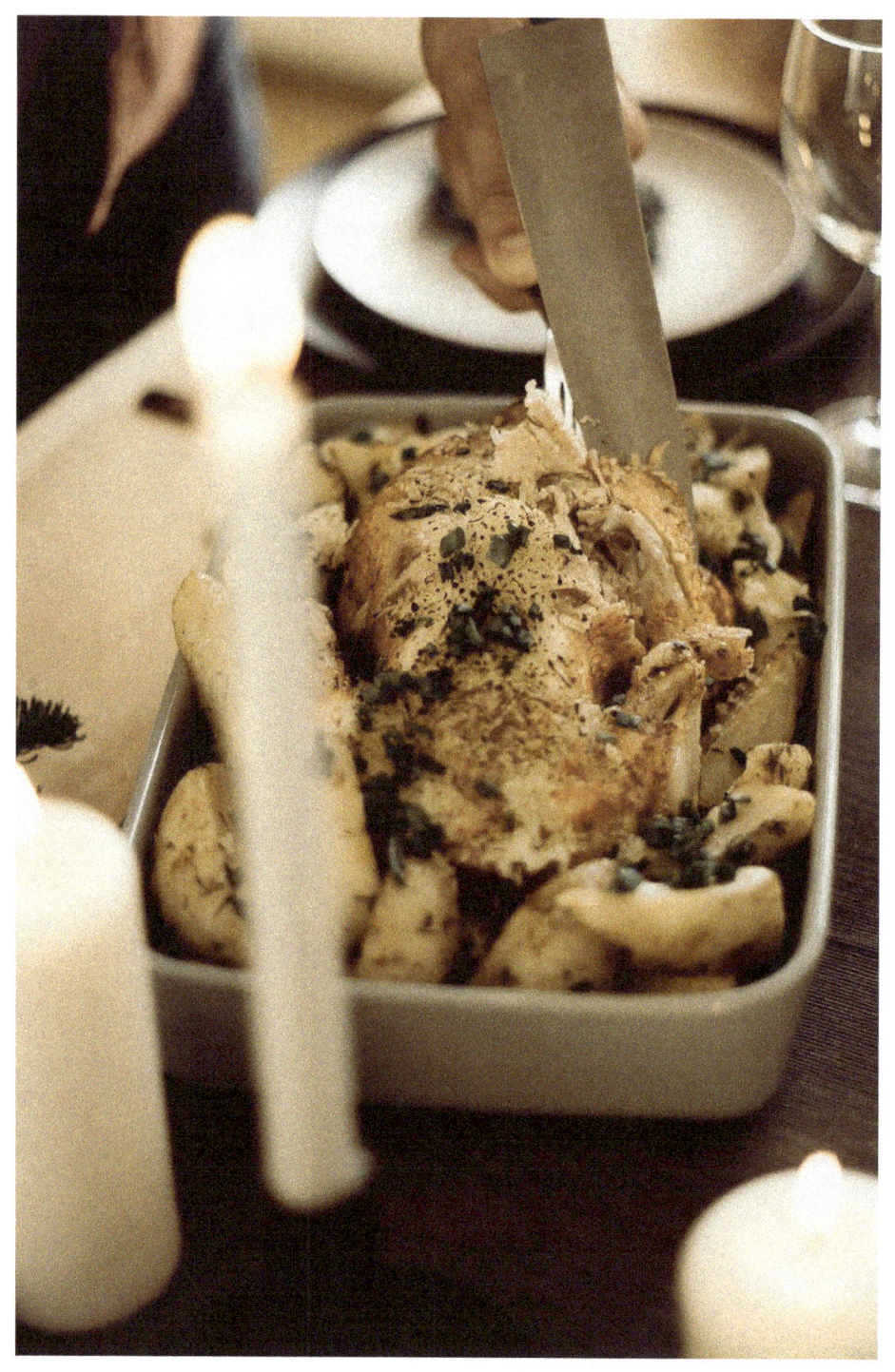

INTRODUCTION

The Keto nutritional regime has always been one of the best and most appreciated!

In this fantastic cookbook we have dedicated ourselves to the most proteinous part of all foods, just poultry.

Chicken has a very high protein intake, with a low amount of fat, so it's perfect for keeping in line but never losing the pleasure of eating delicious dishes.

In this book I have selected the easiest recipes for beginners so that you can train right away. Let's get started right away prepare the kitchen and the apron and enjoy.

POULTRY RECIPES

FESTIVE TURKEY ROULADEN

Ingredients:

- 2 pounds turkey fillet, marinated and cut into 10 pieces

- 10 strips prosciutto

- 1/2 teaspoon chili powder

- 1 teaspoon marjoram

- 1 sprig rosemary, finely chopped

- 2 tablespoons dry white wine

- 1 teaspoon garlic, finely minced

- 1 ½ tablespoons butter, room temperature

- 1 tablespoon Dijon mustard

- Sea salt and freshly ground black pepper, to your liking

Instructions

1. Start by preheating your oven to 430 degrees F.

2. Pat the turkey dry and cook in hot butter for about 3 minutes per side. Add in the mustard, chili powder, marjoram, rosemary, wine, and garlic.

3. Continue to cook for 2 minutes more. Wrap each turkey piece into one prosciutto strip and secure with toothpicks.

4. Roast in the preheated oven for about 30 minutes.

Preparation Time: 15 minutes **Servings:** 5

Cooking Time: 30 minutes

Nutrition: 286 Calories 9.7g Fat 6.9g Carbs 39.9g Protein 0.3g Fiber

PAN-FRIED CHORIZO SAUSAGE

Ingredients:

- 16 ounces smoked turkey chorizo

- 1 ½ cups Asiago cheese, grated

- 1 teaspoon oregano

- 1 teaspoon basil

- 1 cup tomato puree

- 4 scallion stalks, chopped

- 1 teaspoon garlic paste

- Sea salt and ground black pepper, to taste

- 1 tablespoon dry sherry

- 1 tablespoon extra-virgin olive oil

- 2 tablespoons fresh coriander, roughly chopped

Instructions

1. Heat the oil in a frying pan over moderately high heat. Now, brown the turkey chorizo, crumbling with a fork for about 5 minutes.

2. Add in the other Ingredients, except for cheese; continue to cook for 10 minutes more or until cooked through.

Preparation Time: 10 minutes **Servings:** 4

Cooking Time: 20 minutes

Nutrition: 330 Calories 17.2g Fat 4.5g Carbs 34.4g Protein 1.6g Fiber

CHINESE BOK CHOY AND TURKEY SOUP

Ingredients:

- 1/2 pound baby Bok choy, sliced into quarters lengthwise
- 2 pounds turkey carcass
- 1 tablespoon olive oil
- 1/2 cup leeks, chopped
- 1 celery rib, chopped
- 2 carrots, sliced
- 6 cups turkey stock
- Himalayan salt and black pepper, to taste

Instructions

1. In a heavy-bottomed pot, heat the olive oil until sizzling. Once hot, sauté the celery, carrots, leek and Bok choy for about 6 minutes.

2. Add the salt, pepper, turkey, and stock; bring to a boil.

3. Turn the heat to simmer. Continue to cook, partially covered, for about 35 minutes.

Preparation Time: 15 minutes **Servings:** 8

Cooking Time: 40 minutes

Nutrition: 211 Calories 11.8g Fat 3.1g Carbs 23.7g Protein 0.9g Fiber

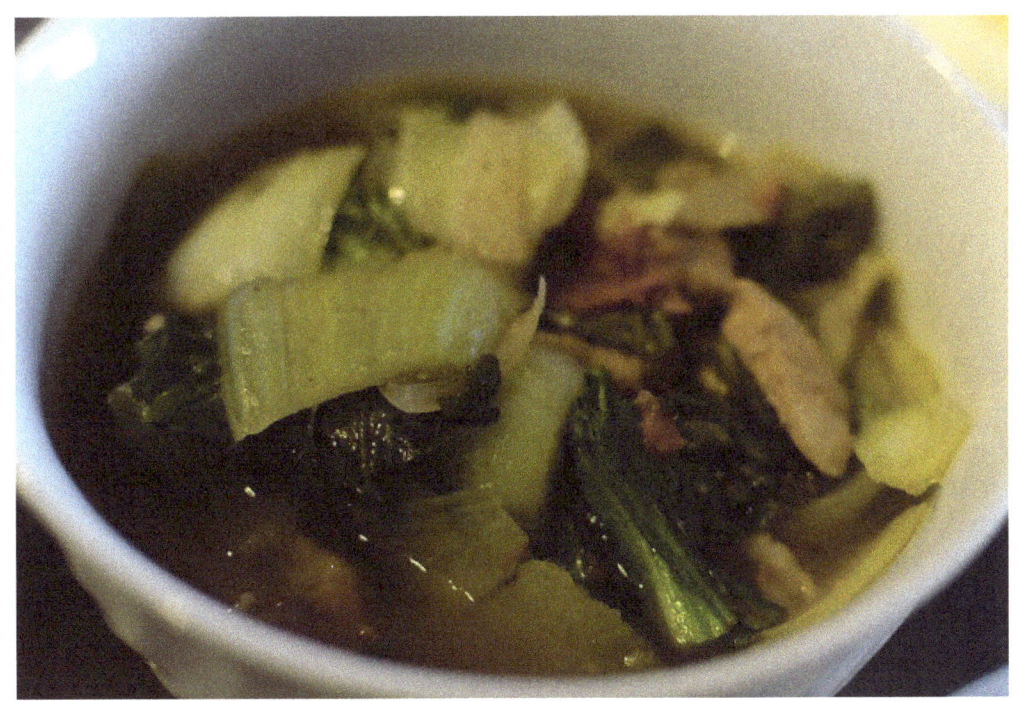

HERBY CHICKEN MEATLOAF

Ingredients:

- 2 ½ lb. ground chicken
- 3 tbsp. flaxseed meal
- 2 large eggs
- 2 tbsp. olive oil
- 1 lemon,1 tbsp. juiced
- ¼ cup chopped parsley
- ¼ cup chopped oregano
- 4 garlic cloves, minced
- Lemon slices to garnish

Instructions

- Preheat oven to 400 F. In a bowl, combine ground chicken and flaxseed meal; set aside. In a small bowl, whisk the eggs with olive oil, lemon juice, parsley, oregano, and garlic.

- Pour the mixture onto the chicken mixture and mix well. Spoon into a greased loaf pan and press to fit. Bake for 40 minutes.

- Remove the pan, drain the liquid, and let cool a bit. Slice, garnish with lemon slices, and serve.

Preparation Time: 20 minutes **Servings:** 6

Cooking Time: 30 minutes

Nutrition: Cal 362 Net Carbs 1.3g Fat 24g Protein 35g

LOVELY PULLED CHICKEN EGG BITES

Ingredients:

- 2 tbsp. butter

- 1 chicken breast

- 2 tbsp. chopped green onions

- ½ tsp red chili flakes

- 12 eggs

- ¼ cup grated Monterey Jack

Instructions

1. Preheat oven to 400 F. Line a 12-hole muffin tin with cupcake liners. Melt butter in a skillet over medium heat and cook the chicken until brown on each side, 10 minutes.

2. Transfer to a plate and shred with 2 forks. Divide between muffin holes along with green onions and red chili flakes.

3. Crack an egg into each muffin hole and scatter the cheese on top. Bake for 15 minutes until eggs set. Serve.

Preparation Time: 15 minutes **Servings:** 4

Cooking Time: 30 minutes

Nutrition: Cal 393 Net Carbs 0.5g Fat 27g Protein 34g

CREAMY MUSTARD CHICKEN WITH SHIRATAKI

Ingredients:

- 2 (8 oz.) packs angel hair shirataki
- 4 chicken breasts, cut into strips
- 1 cup chopped mustard greens
- 1 yellow bell pepper, sliced
- 1 tbsp. olive oil
- 1 yellow onion, finely sliced
- 1 garlic clove, minced
- 1 tbsp. wholegrain mustard
- 5 tbsp. heavy cream
- 1 tbsp. chopped parsley

Instructions

1. Boil 2 cups of water in a medium pot.

2. Strain the shirataki pasta and rinse well under hot running water. Allow proper draining and pour the shirataki pasta into the boiling water.

3. Cook for 3 minutes and strain again. Place a dry skillet and stir-fry the shirataki pasta until visibly dry, 1-2 minutes; set aside.

4. Heat olive oil in a skillet, season the chicken with salt and pepper and cook for 8-10 minutes; set aside. Stir in onion, bell pepper, and garlic and cook until softened, 5 minutes.

5. Mix in mustard and heavy cream; simmer for 2 minutes and mix in the chicken and mustard greens for 2 minutes. Stir in shirataki pasta, garnish with parsley and serve.

Preparation Time: 20 minutes **Servings:** 4

Cooking Time: 30 minutes

Nutrition: Cal 692 Net Carbs 15g Fats 38g Protein 65g

PARSNIP & BACON CHICKEN BAKE

Ingredients:

- 6 bacon slices, chopped
- 2 tbsp. butter
- ½ lb. parsnips, diced
- 2 tbsp. olive oil
- 1 lb. ground chicken
- 2 tbsp. butter
- 1 cup heavy cream
- 2 oz. cream cheese, softened
- 1 ¼ cups grated Pepper Jack
- ¼ cup chopped scallions

Instructions

1. Preheat oven to 300 F. Put the bacon in a pot and fry it until brown and crispy, 6 minutes; set aside. Melt butter in a skillet and sauté parsnips until softened and lightly browned. Transfer to a greased baking sheet.

2. Heat olive oil in the same pan and cook the chicken until no longer pink, 8 minutes. Spoon onto a plate and set aside too.

3. Add heavy cream, cream cheese, and two-thirds of the Pepper Jack cheese to the pot. Melt the ingredients over medium heat, frequently stirring, 7 minutes.

4. Spread the parsnips on the baking dish, top with chicken, pour the heavy cream mixture over, and scatter bacon and scallions.

5. Sprinkle the remaining cheese on top and bake until the cheese melts and is golden, 30 minutes. Serve warm.

Preparation Time: 10 minutes **Servings:** 4

Cooking Time: 50 minutes

Nutrition: Cal 757 Net Carbs 5.5g Fat 66g Protein 29g

CHICKEN BAKE WITH ONION & PARSNIP

Ingredients:

- 3 parsnips, sliced
- 1 onion, sliced
- 4 garlic cloves, crushed
- 2 tbsp. olive oil
- 2 lb. chicken breasts
- ½ cup chicken broth
- ¼ cup white wine
- Salt and black pepper to taste

Instructions

1. Preheat oven to 360 F. Warm oil in a skillet over medium heat and brown chicken for a couple of minutes, and transfer to a baking dish.

2. Arrange the vegetables around the chicken and add in wine and chicken broth. Bake for 25 minutes, stirring once. Serve warm.

Preparation Time: 15 minutes

Cooking Time: 30 minutes

Nutrition: Cal 278 Net Carbs 5.1g Fat 8.7g Protein 35g

CUCUMBER-TURKEY CANAPES

Ingredients:

- 2 cucumbers, sliced
- 2 cups dices leftover turkey
- ¼ jalapeño pepper, minced
- 1 tbsp. Dijon mustard
- ¼ cup mayonnaise
- Salt and black pepper to taste

Instructions

1. Cut mid-level holes in cucumber slices with a knife and set aside.
2. Mix turkey, jalapeno pepper, mustard, mayonnaise, salt, and black pepper in a bowl.
3. Carefully fill cucumber holes with turkey mixture and serve.

Preparation Time: 10 minutes **Servings:** 6

Cooking Time: 5 minutes

Nutrition: Cal 170 Net Carbs 1.3g Fat 14g Protein 10g

BAKED CHICKEN SKEWERS WITH RUTABAGA FRIES

Ingredients:

- 2 chicken breasts, halved

- Salt and black pepper to taste

- 4 tbsp. olive oil

- ¼ cup chicken broth

- 1 lb. rutabaga

- 2 tbsp. olive oil

Instructions

1. Set oven to 400 F. Grease and line a baking sheet. In a bowl, mix 2 tbsp. of the olive oil, salt, and pepper and add in the chicken; toss to coat. Set in the fridge for 20 minutes.

2. Peel and chop rutabaga to form fry shapes and place into a separate bowl. Coat with the remaining olive oil and season with salt and pepper. Arrange the rutabaga shapes on the baking sheet and bake for 10 minutes.

3. Take the chicken from the refrigerator and thread onto the skewers. Place over the rutabaga, pour in the chicken broth, and bake for 30 minutes. Serve immediately.

Preparation Time: 20 minutes **Servings:** 6

Cooking Time: 45 minutes

Nutrition: Cal: 579 Net Carbs: 6g Fat: 53g Protein: 39g

LOUISIANA CHICKEN FETTUCCINE

Ingredients:

- 1 medium red bell pepper, deseeded and thinly sliced
- 1 medium green bell pepper, deseeded and thinly sliced
- 2 cups grated mozzarella
- ½ cup grated Parmesan
- 1 cup shredded mozzarella
- 1 egg yolk
- 2 tbsp. olive oil
- 4 chicken breasts, cubed
- 1 yellow onion, thinly sliced
- 4 garlic cloves, minced
- 4 tsp Cajun seasoning
- 1 cup Alfredo sauce

- ½ cup marinara sauce

- 2 tbsp. chopped fresh parsley

Instructions

1. Microwave mozzarella cheese for 2 minutes. Take out the bowl and allow cooling for 1 minute.

2. Mix in egg yolk until well-combined. Lay a parchment paper on a flat surface, pour the cheese mixture on top and cover with another parchment paper.

3. Flatten the dough into 1/8-inch thickness. Take off the parchment paper and cut the dough into thick fettuccine strands. Place in a bowl and refrigerate overnight.

4. Bring 2 cups water to a boil and add fettuccine. Cook for 1 minute and drain; set aside.

5. Preheat oven to 350 F. Heat olive oil in a skillet and cook chicken for 6 minutes. Transfer to a plate. Add onion, garlic and bell peppers to the skillet and cook for 5 minutes. Return the chicken to the pot and stir in Cajun seasoning, Alfredo sauce, and marinara sauce.

6. Cook for 3 minutes. Stir in fettuccine and transfer to a greased baking dish. Cover with the mozzarella and Parmesan cheeses and bake for 15 minutes. Garnish with parsley and serve.

Preparation Time: 10 minutes **Servings:** 4

Cooking Time: 45 minutes

Nutrition: Cal 778 Net Carbs 4g Fats 38g Protein 93g

CHICKEN WRAPS IN BACON WITH SPINACH

Ingredients:

- 4 chicken breasts

- 8 slices bacon

- Salt and black pepper to taste

- 2 tbsp. olive oil

For the buttered spinach:

- 2 tbsp. butter

- 1 lb. spinach

- 4 garlic cloves, minced

Instructions

1. Preheat oven to 450 F. Wrap each chicken breast with 2 bacon slices, season with salt and pepper, and place on a baking sheet.

2. Drizzle with olive oil and bake for 15 minutes until the bacon browns and chicken cooks within. Melt butter in a skillet and sauté spinach and garlic until the leaves wilt, 5 minutes. Season with salt and pepper.

3. Remove from the oven and serve with buttered spinach.

Preparation Time: 12 minutes **Servings:** 5

Cooking Time: 30 minutes

Nutrition: Cal 856 Net Carbs 2.4g Fat 60g Protein 71g

373. CAULI RICE & CHICKEN COLLARD WRAPS

Ingredients:

- 2 tbsp. avocado oil

- 1 large yellow onion, chopped

- 2 garlic cloves, minced

- Salt and black pepper to taste

- 1 jalapeño pepper, chopped

- 1 ½ lb. chicken breasts, cubed

- 1 cup cauliflower rice

- 2 tsp hot sauce

- 8 collard leaves

- ¼ cup crème fraiche

Instructions

1. Heat avocado oil in a deep skillet and sauté onion and garlic until softened, 3 minutes. Stir in jalapeño pepper salt, and pepper.

2. Mix in chicken and cook until no longer pink on all sides, 10 minutes. Add in cauliflower rice and hot sauce. Sauté until the cauliflower slightly softens, 3 minutes.

3. Lay out the collards on a clean flat surface and spoon the curried mixture onto the middle part of the leaves, about 3 tbsp. per leaf. Spoon crème fraiche on top, wrap the leaves, and serve immediately.

Preparation Time: 10 minutes **Servings:** 4

Cooking Time: 30 minutes

Nutrition: Cal 437 Net Carbs 1.8g Fat 28g Protein 38g

374. **STUFFED PEPPERS WITH CHICKEN & BROCCOLI**

Ingredients:

- 6 yellow bell peppers, halved
- 1 ½ tbsp. olive oil
- 3 tbsp. butter
- 3 garlic cloves, minced
- ½ white onion, chopped
- 2 lb. ground chicken
- 3 tsp taco seasoning
- 1 cup rice broccoli
- ¼ cup grated cheddar cheese
- Crème fraiche for serving

Instructions

1. Preheat oven to 400 F. Drizzle bell peppers with olive oil. Melt butter in a skillet and sauté garlic and onion for 3 minutes.

2. Stir in chicken and taco seasoning. Cook for 8 minutes. Mix in broccoli. Spoon the mixture into the peppers, top with cheddar cheese, and place in a greased baking dish.

3. Bake until the cheese melts and is bubbly, 30 minutes. Top with the crème fraiche and serve.

Preparation Time: 35 minutes **Servings:** 6

Cooking Time: 2 hours

Nutrition: Cal 386 Net Carbs 11g Fat 24g Protein 30g

GRILLED CHICKEN KEBABS WITH CURRY & YOGURT

Ingredients:

- 1 ½ lb. boneless chicken thighs, cut into 1-inch pieces

- ½ cup Greek yogurt

- Salt and black pepper to taste

- 2 tbsp. curry powder

- 1 tbsp. olive oil

Instructions

1. Preheat oven to 380 F. In a bowl, combine Greek yogurt, salt, pepper, curry, and olive oil. Mix in chicken, cover the bowl with a plastic wrap and marinate for 20 minutes.

2. Remove the wrap and thread the chicken onto skewers. Grill in the middle rack of the oven for 4 minutes on each side or until fully cooked.

3. Remove the chicken skewers and serve with cauliflower rice or steamed green beans.

Preparation Time: 10 minutes **Servings:** 4

Cooking Time: 15 minutes

Nutrition: Cal 440 Net Carbs 0.5g Fat 29g Protein 41g

CHICKEN WITH TOMATO AND ZUCCHINI

Ingredients:

- 2 tbsp. ghee
- 1 lb. chicken thighs
- 2 cloves garlic, minced
- 1 (14 oz.) can whole tomatoes
- 1 zucchini, diced
- 10 fresh basil leaves, chopped

Instructions

1. Melt ghee in a saucepan and fry chicken for 4 minutes on each side. Remove to a plate. Sauté garlic in the same saucepan for 2 minutes, pour in tomatoes, and cook for 8 minutes.

2. Add in zucchini and cook for 4 minutes. Stir and add the chicken. Coat with sauce and simmer for 3 minutes. Serve chicken with sauce garnished with basil.

Preparation Time: 10 minutes **Servings:** 4

Cooking Time: 45 minutes

Nutrition: Cal 468 Net Carbs 2g Fat 39g Protein 26g

CREAM CHEESE & TURKEY PASTRAMI ROLLS

Ingredients:

- 10 canned pepperoncini peppers, sliced and drained
- 8 oz. softened cream cheese
- 10 oz. turkey pastrami, sliced

Instructions

1. Lay a plastic wrap on a flat surface and arrange the pastrami all over, slightly overlapping each other. Spread the cheese on top of the salami and arrange the pepperoncini on top.

2. Hold 2 opposite ends of the plastic wrap and roll the pastrami.

3. Twist both ends to tighten and refrigerate for 2 hours. Slice into 2-inch pinwheels. Serve.

Preparation Time: 20 minutes **Servings:** 4

Cooking Time: 2 hours 40 minutes

Nutrition: Cal 266 Net Carbs 1g Fat 24g Protein 13g

ALMOND CRUSTED CHICKEN ZUCCHINI STACKS

Ingredients:

- 1 ½ lb. chicken thighs, skinless and boneless, cut into strips
- 3 tbsp. almond flour
- Salt and black pepper to taste
- 2 large zucchinis, sliced
- 4 tbsp. olive oil
- 2 tsp Italian mixed herb blend
- ½ cup chicken broth

Instructions

1. Preheat oven to 400 F. In a zipper bag, add almond flour, salt, and pepper. Mix and add the chicken strips. Seal the bag and shake to coat.

2. Arrange the zucchinis on a greased baking sheet. Season with salt and pepper and drizzle with 2 tbsp. of olive oil.

3. Remove the chicken from the almond flour mixture, shake off, and put 2-3 chicken strips on each zucchini.

4. Season with herb blend and drizzle again with the remaining olive oil. Bake for 8 minutes; then pour in broth. Bake further for 10 minutes. Serve warm.

Preparation Time: 20 minutes **Servings:** 4

Cooking Time: 30 minutes

Nutrition: Cal 512 Net Carbs 1.2g Fat 42g Protein 29g

PALEO COCONUT FLOUR CHICKEN NUGGETS

Ingredients:

- ½ cup coconut flour

- 1 egg

- 2 tbsp. garlic powder

- 2 chicken breasts, cubed

- Salt and black pepper, to taste

- ½ cup butter

Instructions

1. In a bowl, combine salt, garlic powder, flour, and pepper and stir. In a separate bowl, beat the egg. Add the chicken in egg mixture, then in the flour mixture.

2. Set a pan over medium heat and warm butter. Add in chicken nuggets, and cook for 6 minutes on each side.

3. Remove to paper towels, drain the excess grease, and serve.

Preparation Time: 10 minutes **Servings:** 2

Cooking Time: 30 minutes

Nutrition: Cal 417 Net Carbs 4.3g Fat 37g Protein 35g

CHICKEN FAJITA BOWLS

Ingredients:

- 1 pound (454 g) boneless, skinless chicken breasts, cut into 1-inch pieces

- 2 cups chicken broth

- 1 cup salsa

- 1 teaspoon paprika

- 1 teaspoon fine sea salt, or more to taste

- 1 teaspoon chili powder

- ½ teaspoon ground cumin

- ½ teaspoon ground black pepper

- 1 lime, halved

Instructions

1. Combine all the ingredients except the lime in the Instant Pot.

2. Lock the cover. Select the Manual mode and adjust the cooking time for ten minutes at a very High Pressure.

3. When the timer beeps, perform a quick pressure release. Carefully remove the lid.

4. Shred the chicken with two forks and return to the Instant Pot. Squeeze the lime juice into the chicken mixture. Taste and add more salt, if needed. Give the mixture a good stir.

5. Ladle the chicken mixture into bowls and serve.

Preparation Time: 5 minutes **Servings:** 2

Cooking Time: 10 minutes

Nutrition: calories: 281 fat: 6.3g protein: 51.5g carbs: 5.9g net carbs: 4.9g fiber: 1.0g

PROSCIUTTO-WRAPPED CHICKEN

Ingredients:

- 1½ cups water

- 5 chicken breast halves, butterflied

- 2 garlic cloves, halved

- 1 teaspoon marjoram

- Sea salt, to taste

- ½ teaspoon red pepper flakes

- ¼ teaspoon ground black pepper, or more to taste

- 10 strips prosciutto

Instructions

1. Pour the water into the Instant Pot and insert the trivet.

2. Rub the chicken breast halves with garlic. Sprinkle with marjoram, salt, red pepper flakes, and black pepper. Wrap

each chicken breast into 2 prosciutto strips and secure with toothpicks. Put the chicken on the trivet.

3. Lock the lid. Select the Poultry mode and set the cooking time for 15 minutes at High Pressure.

4. When the timer beeps, perform a natural pressure release for 10 minutes, then release any remaining pressure. Carefully remove the lid.

5. Remove the toothpicks and serve warm.

Preparation Time: 5 minutes **Servings:** 5

Cooking Time: 15 minutes

Nutrition: calories: 550 fat: 28.6g protein: 68.5g carbs: 1.0g net carbs: 0.8g fiber: 0.2g

CREAMY CHICKEN CORDON BLEU

Ingredients:

- 4 boneless, skinless chicken breast halves, butterflied

- 4 (1-ounce / 28-g) slices Swiss cheese

- 8 (1-ounce / 28-g) slices ham

- 1 cup water

- Chopped fresh flat-leaf parsley, for garnish

Sauce:

- 1½ ounces (43 g) cream cheese (3 tablespoons)

- ¼ cup chicken broth

- 1 tablespoon unsalted butter

- ¼ teaspoon ground black pepper

- ¼ teaspoon fine sea salt

Instructions

- Lay the chicken breast halves on a clean work surface. Top each with a slice of Swiss cheese and 2 slices of ham. Roll the chicken around the ham and cheese, then secure with toothpicks. Set aside.

- Whisk together all the ingredients for the sauce in a small saucepan over medium heat, stirring until the cream cheese melts and the sauce is smooth.

- Place the chicken rolls, seam-side down, in a casserole dish. Pour half of the sauce over the chicken rolls. Set the remaining sauce aside.

- Pour the water into the Instant Pot and insert the trivet. Place the dish on the trivet.

- Lock the lid. Select the Manual mode and set the cooking time for 15 minutes at High Pressure.

- When the timer beeps, perform a natural pressure release for 10 minutes, then release any remaining pressure. Carefully remove the lid.

- Remove the chicken rolls from the Instant Pot to a plate. Pour the remaining sauce over them and serve garnished with the parsley.

Preparation Time: 12 minutes **Servings:** 6

Cooking Time: 15 minutes

Nutrition: calories: 314 fat: 13.6g protein: 46.2g carbs: 1.7g net carbs: 1.7g fiber: 0g

CHEESY CHICKEN DRUMSTICKS

Ingredients:

- 1 tablespoon olive oil

- 5 chicken drumsticks

- ½ cup chicken stock

- ¼ cup unsweetened coconut milk

- ¼ cup dry white wine

- 2 garlic cloves, minced

- 1 teaspoon shallot powder

- ½ teaspoon marjoram

- ½ teaspoon thyme

- 6 ounces (170 g) ricotta cheese

- 4 ounces (113 g) Cheddar cheese

- ½ teaspoon cayenne pepper

- ¼ teaspoon ground black pepper

- Sea salt, to taste

Instructions

1. Set your Instant Pot to Sauté and heat the olive oil until sizzling.

2. Add the chicken drumsticks and brown each side for 3 minutes.

3. Stir in the chicken stock, milk, wine, garlic, shallot powder, marjoram, thyme.

4. Lock the lid. Select the Manual mode and set the cooking time for 15 minutes at High Pressure.

5. When the timer beeps, perform a natural pressure release for 10 minutes, then release any remaining pressure. Carefully remove the lid.

6. Shred the chicken with two forks and return to the Instant Pot.

7. Set your Instant Pot to Sauté again and add the remaining ingredients and stir well.

8. Cook for another 2 minutes, or until the cheese is melted. Taste and add more salt, if desired. Serve immediately.

Preparation Time: 3 minutes **Servings:** 5

Cooking Time: 23 minutes

Nutrition: calories: 413 fat: 24.3g protein: 41.9g carbs: 4.6g net carbs: 4.0g fiber: 0.6g

JAMAICAN CURRY CHICKEN DRUMSTICKS

Ingredients:

- 1½ pounds (680 g) chicken drumsticks

- 1 tablespoon Jamaican curry powder

- 1 teaspoon salt

- 1 cup chicken broth

- ½ medium onion, diced

- ½ teaspoon dried thyme

Instructions

- Sprinkle the salt and curry powder over the chicken drumsticks.

- Place the chicken drumsticks into the Instant Pot, along with the remaining ingredients.

- Secure the lid. Select the Manual mode and set the cooking time for 20 minutes at High Pressure.

- Once cooking is done, do a quick pressure release. Open the lid and serve warm.

Preparation Time: 5 minutes **Servings:** 4

Cooking Time: 20 minutes

Nutrition: calories: 290 fat: 14.6g protein: 31.8g carbs: 1.6g net carbs: 1.3g fiber: 0.3g

PARMESAN DRUMSTICKS

Ingredients:

- 2 pounds (907 g) chicken drumsticks (about 8 pieces)

- 1 teaspoon salt

- 1 teaspoon dried parsley

- ½ teaspoon garlic powder

- ½ teaspoon dried oregano

- ¼ teaspoon pepper

- 1 cup water

- 1 stick butter

- 2 ounces (57 g) cream cheese, softened

- ½ cup grated Parmesan cheese

- ½ cup chicken broth

- ¼ cup heavy cream

- 1/8 teaspoon pepper

Instructions

1. Sprinkle the salt, parsley, garlic powder, oregano, and pepper evenly over the chicken drumsticks.

2. Pour the water into the Instant Pot and insert the trivet. Arrange the drumsticks on the trivet.

3. Secure the lid. Select the Manual mode and set the cooking time for 15 minutes at High Pressure.

4. Once cooking is complete, do a quick pressure release. Carefully open the lid.

5. Transfer the drumsticks to a foil-lined baking sheet and broil each side for 3 to 5 minutes, or until the skin begins to crisp.

6. Meanwhile, pour the water out of the Instant Pot. Set your Instant Pot to Sauté and melt the butter.

7. Add the remaining ingredients to the Instant Pot and whisk to combine. Pour the sauce over the drumsticks and serve warm.

Preparation Time: 5 minutes **Servings:** 4

Cooking Time: 25 minutes

Nutrition: calories: 788 fat: 55.8g protein: 53.7g carbs: 3.4g net carbs: 3.3g fiber: 0.1g

CHICKEN LEGS WITH MAYO SAUCE

Ingredients:

- 4 chicken legs, bone-in, skinless
- 2 garlic cloves, peeled and halved
- ½ teaspoon coarse sea salt
- ½ teaspoon crushed red pepper flakes
- ¼ teaspoon ground black pepper, or more to taste
- 1 tablespoon olive oil
- ¼ cup chicken broth

Dipping Sauce:

- ¾ cup mayonnaise
- 2 tablespoons stone ground mustard
- 1 teaspoon fresh lemon juice
- ½ teaspoon Sriracha

For Garnish:

- ¼ cup roughly chopped fresh cilantro

Instructions

1. Rub the chicken legs with the garlic. Sprinkle with salt, red pepper flakes, and black pepper.

2. Set your Instant Pot to Sauté and heat the olive oil.

3. Add the chicken legs and brown for 4 to 5 minutes. Add a splash of chicken broth to deglaze the bottom of the pot.

4. Pour the remaining chicken broth into the Instant Pot and mix well.

5. Lock the lid. Select the Manual mode and set the cooking time for 14 minutes at High Pressure.

6. Meanwhile, whisk together all the sauce ingredients in a small bowl.

7. When the timer beeps, perform a natural pressure release for 10 minutes, then release any remaining pressure. Carefully remove the lid.

8. Sprinkle the cilantro on top for garnish and serve with the prepared dipping sauce.

Preparation Time: 5 minutes **Servings:** 4

Cooking Time: 20 minutes

Nutrition: calories: 487 fat: 42.9g protein: 22.7g carbs: 2.2g net carbs: 1.5g fiber: 0.7g

CHICKEN WITH CHEESE MUSHROOM SAUCE

Ingredients:

- 2 tablespoons unsalted butter or coconut oil
- 2 cloves garlic, minced
- ¼ cup diced onions
- 2 cups sliced button or cremini mushrooms
- 4 boneless, skinless chicken breast halves
- ½ cup chicken broth
- ¼ cup heavy cream
- 1 teaspoon fine sea salt
- 1 teaspoon dried tarragon leaves
- ½ teaspoon dried thyme leaves
- ½ teaspoon ground black pepper
- 2 bay leaves

- ½ cup grated Parmesan cheese

- Fresh thyme leaves, for garnish

Instructions

- Set your Instant Pot to Sauté and melt the butter.

- Add the garlic, onions, and mushrooms and sauté for 4 minutes, stirring often, or until the onions are softened.

- Add the remaining ingredients except the Parmesan cheese and thyme leaves to the Instant Pot and stir to combine.

- Seal the lid. Select Manual mode then set the cooking time for ten minutes at High Pressure.

- When the timer beeps, perform a natural pressure release for 10 minutes, then release any remaining pressure. Carefully remove the lid.

- Discard the bay leaves and transfer the chicken to a serving platter.

- Add the Parmesan cheese to the Instant Pot with the sauce and stir until the cheese melts.

- Pour the mushroom sauce from the pot over the chicken. Serve garnished with the fresh thyme leaves.

Preparation Time: 8 minutes **Servings:** 4

Cooking Time: 14 minutes

Nutrition: calories: 278 fat: 17.3g protein: 27.5g carbs: 5.1g net carbs: 4.1g fiber: 1.0g

CHICKEN CACCIATORE

Ingredients:

- 6 tablespoons coconut oil

- 5 chicken legs

- 1 bell pepper, diced

- ½ onion, chopped

- 1 (14-ounce / 397-g) can sugar-free or low-sugar diced tomatoes

- ½ teaspoon dried basil

- ½ teaspoon dried parsley

- ½ teaspoon kosher salt

- ½ teaspoon freshly ground black pepper

- ½ cup filtered water

Instructions

1. Press the Sauté button on the Instant Pot and melt the coconut oil.

2. Add the chicken legs and sauté until the outside is browned.

3. Remove the chicken and set aside.

4. Add the bell pepper, onion, tomatoes, basil, parsley, salt, and pepper to the Instant Pot and cook for about 2 minutes.

5. Pour in the water and return the chicken to the pot.

6. Lock the lid. Select the Manual mode and set the cooking time for 18 minutes at High Pressure.

7. Once cooking is complete, carefully open the lid. Serve warm.

Preparation Time: 5 minutes **Servings:** 4 to 5

Cooking Time: 22 minutes

Nutrition: calories: 346 fat: 24.5g protein: 26.8g carbs: 5.0g net carbs: 3.4g fiber: 1.6g

SALSA CHICKEN LEGS

Ingredients:

- 5 chicken legs, skinless and boneless
- ½ teaspoon sea salt

Salsa Sauce:

- 1 cup puréed tomatoes
- 1 cup onion, chopped
- 1 jalapeño, chopped
- 2 bell peppers, deveined and chopped
- 2 tablespoons minced fresh cilantro
- 3 teaspoons lime juice
- 1 teaspoon granulated garlic

Instructions

1. Press the Sauté button to heat your Instant Pot.

2. Add the chicken legs and sear each side for 2 to 3 minutes until evenly browned. Season with sea salt.

3. Thoroughly combine all the ingredients for the salsa sauce in a mixing bowl. Spoon the salsa mixture evenly over the browned chicken legs.

4. Seal the Cover. Fix the Manual mode and put the cooking time for 10 minutes at High Pressure.

5. When the timer beeps, perform a natural pressure release for 10 minutes, then release any remaining pressure. Carefully remove the lid. Serve warm.

Preparation Time: 5 minutes **Servings:** 5

Cooking Time: 16 minutes

Nutrition: calories: 357 fat: 11.6g protein: 52.4g carbs: 8.6g net carbs: 7.0g fiber: 1.6g

DESSERT RECIPES

PEANUT BUTTER CHOCOLATE CAKE

Ingredients

8. 15.25 oz devil eat cake mix

9. 1 cup water

10. ½ cup melted salted butter

11. 3 eggs

12. 8 oz Package of Mini Reese's Peanut Butter Cups

13. 1 cup creamy peanut butter

14. 3 caster sugar tsp

15. Ten Reese's peanut butter cups

Instructions

1. In a large bowl, combine the cake mix, ice cream, butter, and eggs until smooth. Cut the mini peanut butter cups.

2. Melt butter in the pan and spread evenly.

3. Cover and cook on high for 2 hours.

4. Place the peanut butter in a small saucepan on the stove over medium heat. Stir until it is melted and smooth. Add the powdered sugar and beat to soften.

Prep time: 15 min; **Servings:** 10

Macros: Cal 607, Carbs 57 g, Protein 13 g, Fat 39 g, Saturated Fat 13 g

CROCKPOT APPLE PUDDING CAKE

Ingredients

4. 2 cups all-purpose flour

5. 2/3 cup plus ¼ cup divided sugar

6. 3 tsp of baking soda

7. 1 tsp salt

8. ½ cup cold butter

9. 1 cup milk

10. 4 apples, peeled and diced

11. 1 ½ cup orange juice

12. ½ cup honey or brown sugar

13. 2 Tbsp melted butter

14. 1 tsp cinnamon

Instructions

1. Combine flour, 2/3 cup sugar, baking powder, and salt. Cut the butter until you have thick crumbs in the mixture.

2. Remove the milk from the crumbs until it becomes moist.

3. Grease the bottom and sides of a 4 or 5-liter slow cooker. Place the dough at the bottom of the pot and spread it evenly.

4. Beat the orange juice, honey, butter, remaining sugar and cinnamon in a medium pan. Decorate the apples.

5. Place the jar opening with a clean cloth, place the lid. Prevents condensation on the cover from reaching the pot. Place the pan on top and cook until apples are tender for 2 to 3 hours.

Prep time: 20 min; **Servings:** 10

Macros: Cal 405 Fat 9 g Saturated fat 3 g Carbs 79 g Fiber 2 g Sugar 63 g Protein 3 g

BROWNIE COOKIES

Ingredients

- A box of brownie mix

- 2 eggs

- ¼ cup melted butter, ½ cup mini chocolate chips

- ½ c optional chopped nuts

- 8 slices of cookie dough or spoons filled with a bathtub

Instructions

1. If desired, combine your brownie mix with butter, eggs, chocolate chips, and nuts.

2. Sprinkle the inside of your slow cooker with a non-stick spray.

3. Place 8 slices of prepared cookie dough at the bottom.

4. Pour the brownie mixture into your slow cooker and smooth it evenly.

5. Put the lid on and cook for 2 hours.

Prep time: 15 min; **Servings:** 10

Macros: 452 Cal, 21 g fat, 7 g saturated fat, 59 g Carbs, 38 g sugar, 5 g protein

CHOCOLATE CARAMEL MONKEY BREAD

Ingredients

4. ½ Tbsp sugar

5. ¼ tsp ground cinnamon

6. 15 oz whey cookies

7. 20 candies coated with milk chocolate

8. caramel sauce to cover (optional)

9. chocolate sauce to include (optional)

Instructions

1. Mix sugar and cinnamon and set aside.

2. Fill a jar with parchment paper, cover to the bottom.

3. Wrap 1 buttermilk cookie dough around a chocolate candy to completely cover the candy and close the seam. Place the candy wrapped in cookies at the bottom of the jar, start in the middle of the pot and continue on the side.

4. Continue to wrap the candies and place them in the slow cooker, leaving about ½ inch between each. Repeat these steps with sweets wrapped in the second layer of cookies. Sprinkle the rest of the sugar and cinnamon mixture over the dough.

5. Cover the pan and cook for 1 hour 30 min. After cooking, remove the cover and allow it to cool slightly. Use the edges of the parchment paper to lift the monkey bread from the jar and move it onto a wire rack. Let cool for at least 10-15 min

6. Cut off the excess baking paper around the edge when you're ready to serve. Place the monkey bread in a shallow pan or bowl and sprinkle with chocolate sauce and caramel sauce.

Prep time: 10 min; **Servings:** 6

Macros: Cal 337k saturated fat 16g Carbs 44g Fiber 1g Sugar 12g Protein 5g

COFFEE CAKE

Ingredients

- 2 ½ cups all-purpose flour

- 1 ½ cups packed brown sugar

- 2/3 cups vegetable oil

- 1 ⅓ cups almond milk

- 2 tsp of baking soda

- ½ tsp of baking soda

- 1 tsp ground cinnamon

- 1 tsp white vinegar

- 1 tsp salt

- 2 eggs

- ½ cup optional chopped nuts

Instructions

- Beat flour, brown sugar, and salt in a large bowl. Add the oil until it is crumbly.

- Mix baking powder, baking powder, and cinnamon with a wooden spoon or spatula in the flour mixture. Place the milk, oil, eggs, and vinegar in a measuring cup and mix until the eggs are crushed, add them to the flour mixture and stir until they are combined (the dough may be slightly lumpy).

- Spray a 5-7Q non-stick cooking spray or a line with a slow cooking spray. Pour into the pot with the dough.

- Sprinkle nuts over the cake dough at the end.

- Place a large paper towel over the insert and place the lid on it. Cook over high heat for 1 ½ to 2 ½ hours or until a toothpick is used to clean the edges. The middle is perhaps a little poorly done at the top.

- Serve hot directly from the slow cooker or keep up to 3 days in an airtight container. Use the slow cooker liner to serve effectively. You can lift the whole box, peel it off, and help the cake this way.

- Use a 9 x 13-inch pan sprayed with non-stick cooking oil in a conventional oven and bake for about 35 to 45 min

Prep time: 10 min; **Servings:** 10 to 12

Macro Cal 411, Carbs 56 g, Protein 6g, Fat 19 g Saturated Fat 3g, Fiber 2g, Sugar 33 g

SLOW-COOKING APPLE PEAR CRISP

Ingredients

- 4 apples, peeled and sliced ½ inch

- 3 pears, peeled and sliced ½ inch

- ⅓ cup light brown sugar

- 1 Tbsp flour

- 1 Tbsp lemon juice

- ½ tsp ground cinnamon

- ¼ tsp kosher salt

- A pinch of ground nutmeg

- For the icing

- 3/4 cup all-purpose flour

- 3/4 cup rolled oats

- ½ cup chopped nuts

- ⅓ cup light brown sugar

- ½ tsp ground cinnamon

- ½ tsp kosher salt

- 8 Tbsp unsalted butter, diced

Instructions

1. Combine flour, oats, nuts, sugar, cinnamon, and salt to make the dressing. Use your hands to press the butter into the dry ingredients until it looks like thick crumbs; set aside.

2. Lightly cover with a nonstick spray in a 4-quart slow cooker: put the apples and pears in the slow cooker. Add brown sugar, flour, lemon juice, cinnamon, salt, and nutmeg. Gently press the crumbs into the butter with your fingertips.

3. Place the slow cooker with a clean cloth. Cover and cook for 2 to 3 hours on low heat or for 90 min at high temperature, remove the fabric and continue cooking uncovered until the top is brown and the apples are tender for about 1 hour.

4. Serve cold.

Prep time: 15 min; **Servings:** 8

Macros: Cal 267 | Carbs 27 g | Protein 3g | Fat 17 g | Saturated Fat 7 g | Fiber 4 g | Sugar 16 g

PERFECT CHEESECAKE

Ingredients

For the dough:

- 1 ½ cups graham cracker crumbs

- 6 Tbsp melted butter

For the cheesecake filling:

- 24 g of cream cheese

- 1 ½ cups sour cream

- 1 ¼ cups granulated sugar

- 5 large eggs

- 3 Tbsp all-purpose flour

- 1 Tbsp vanilla extract

- ½ tsp salt

Instructions

1. Light oval 6-quart slow cooker. Place a large piece of baking paper at the bottom of the pan and cover it with a non-stick coating. Place the Graham crackers in a food processor to make crumbs. Then for the milk and pump to mix again. Pour the crumbs into the barrel and press evenly on the bottom.

2. Remove the bowl from the food processor and add the cream cheese and sugar. For a soft wrist. Scrape, add sour cream, eggs, flour, vanilla, and salt. Puree to very mild.

3. For the filling over the crust. Cover the pan and cook slowly for 5-7 hours until a skewer in the middle comes out clean. Remove the moisture from the lid so that it does not drip onto the cheesecake.

4. Place the jar in the refrigerator for at least 3 hours and allow it to cool. Carefully pass all cheesecakes through the edges of the bowl paper. Peel, cut, and serve the paperback!

Prep time: 10 min; **Presentation:** - 20

Macros: Cal 278 , Carbs 20 g, Protein 4 g, Fat 20 g, saturated Fat 11 g, Sugar 15 g

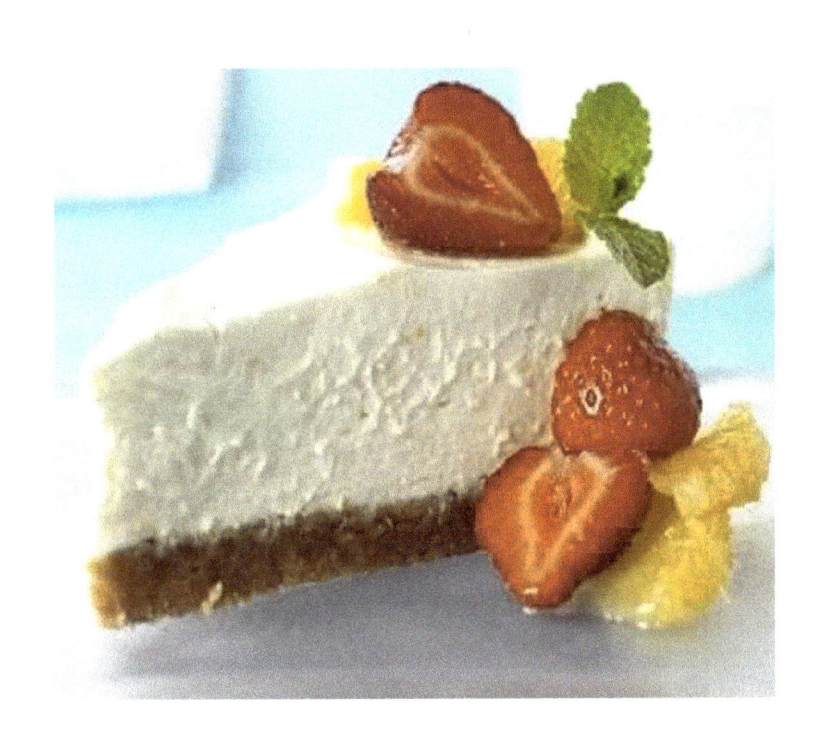

SLOW COOKING LEMON PASTRY

Ingredients

- 1 3/4 cup flour

- ½ cup yellow corn flour

- 3/4 cup butter, sweet

- 1 ¼ cup sugar

- 1 cup sour cream

- 1 cup caster sugar

- 2 eggs

- Tbsp lemon zest, tsp vanilla extract, 1 ½ tsp poppy seeds, 2 ½ Tbsp lemon juice, a tsp bicarbonate soda, 1 tsp of baking soda, ½ tsp salt

Instructions

1. Cover a slow cooker with lightly greased baking paper, 6 liters.

2. Combine flour, cornflour, baking powder, baking powder, and salt in a medium bowl. Put aside.

3. Beat the butter and sugar with an electric mixer until smooth, about 2 min

4. Add the eggs and beat for another 2 min

5. Mix the sour cream, lemon zest, vanilla extract, and poppy seeds with the mixer on low heat.

6. Add the flour mixture slowly and mix well.

7. Pour the dough into the slow cooker with baking paper for 2 hours, 15 min to 2 hours and 30 min, cover, and cook hot. The cake should be placed in the center.

8. Remove the cover and turn off the slow cooker.

9. In a small bowl, beat the lemon juice and powdered sugar.

10. It's okay. Remove it from the insert and place it on a cooling rack. Spray the lemon/sugar mixture on top.

Presentation: – 6; **Prep time:** 10 min

KEY LIME DUMP CAKE

Ingredients

- 15.25 oz Betty Crocker French Vanilla Cake Mix Box

- 44 oz Filled with lime cake {2 boxes of 22 oz Each}

- 8 Tbsp or ½ cup melted butter {1 stick}

Instructions

1. Spray the inside of the clay pot with a non-stick cooking spray. Empty lime cake pans fill the bottom of the clay pot and distribute it evenly.

2. Mix the dried vanilla cake mix with the melted butter in a large bowl and stir until it crumbles. Break the large pieces into small pieces of spoon}.

3. Pour the cake / crumbled butter mixture over the lime jar mixture, spread it evenly, and cover the jar with the lid.

4. Cook 2 hours HIGH or 4 hours DOWN.

5. Serve with ice cream or whipped cream and TASTE.

Prep time: 20 min; **Servings:** 8

Macros: Cal 280 | Carbs 58 g | Protein 2g | Fat 4 g Saturated Fat 2g | Sugar 41 g |

CROCKPOT CANDY SAUCE

Ingredients

- 28 oz sweet condensed milk

- 4 glass jars with full mouth {8 oz each}

Instructions

3. For sweetened condensed milk evenly into 4 containers, leaving 1 " of space at the top of each box.

4. Solid screw caps.

5. Place the jars in the Crockpot and fill the Crockpot with lukewarm water until the jars are completely submerged, with about 1 " of additional water on the bottle caps.

6. Cook 9 hours over LOW heat.

7. Carefully remove the jars with tweezers after 9 hours and allow them to cool for 30 min

8. Once the jars have cooled, remove the lids, take the apple slices and dip in your delicious caramel sauce.

Prep time: 5 min; **Servings:** 4

Macros: Cal 91 | Carbs 15 g | Protein 2g | Fat 2 g Saturated Fat 1 g | Potassium 105 mg | Sugar 15 g

CHERRY PASTRY CROCKPOT

Ingredients

- 15.25 oz Betty Crocker's Devil Cake Mix

- 42 oz Cherry pie filling {2 boxes of 21 oz Each}

- ½ cup melted butter {8 Tbsp. or 113 g}

Instructions

1. Spray nonstick cooking spray

2. 2 in the slow cooker.

3. Empty the cherry pie pans at the bottom of the Crockpot and distribute them evenly.

4. Mix the dry cake mix with melted butter in a medium bowl and stir until it crumbles. Break large pieces into small pieces of spoon}.

5. Pour the cake/butter mixture over the Crockpot cherries, spread it evenly, and cover the Crockpot with a lid.

6. Cook 2 hours HIGH or 4 hours DOWN. Use an ice cream or whipped cream to serve.

7. ENJOY !!

Prep time: 5 min; **Servings:** 8

Macros: 566 Cal, 17 g fat, 11 g saturated fat, 98 g Carbs, 1 g fiber, 37 g sugar, 3 g protein

CROCKPOT PUMPKIN CAKE

Ingredients

- 15.25 oz Betty Crocker Spice Cake Mix {1 Box}

- 15 oz Libby Pure Pumpkin {1 box}

- ½ cup apple sauce

- 3 eggs

- 1 tsp pumpkin pie with herbs

Instructions

5. Beat all the ingredients with a blender for 1 minute.

6. Spray nonstick coating into the slow cooker.

7. Pour and cover the mixture in the Crockpot.

8. Bake for 1.5 to 2 hours or until cooked through.

9. I do not carefully cut the pieces directly from Crock Pot until after the cake is made.

Prep time: 5 min; **Servings:** 8

Macros: Total CARBONS NET 4.42 g, Cal 344, Fat 30.38 g, Carbs 10.03 g, Fiber 5.61 g, Protein 8.26 g

BLUEBERRY CAKE

Ingredients

- 15.25 oz Betty Crocker Lemon Cake Mix {1 box}

- 42 oz Filled with blueberry pie {2 boxes of 21 oz Each}

- ½ cup melted butter {8 Tbsp}

Instructions

1. Spray with a non-stick cooking spray.

2. The crock pot is back. Blueberry pie Fills the empty boxes and distributes them evenly at the bottom of the Crockpot.

3. Mix the dry lemon cake mixture in a mixing bowl with melted butter and stir until it crumbles. Break large pieces into the crumbs of a small spoon.

4. For the cake and butter mixture over the cranberry mixture in Crockpot, spread it evenly and cover the jar with a lid.

5. Cook HIGH for 2 hours and LOW for 4 hours.

6. Serve with ENJOY ice cream and whipped cream !!

Prep time: 5 min; **Servings:** 8

Macros: Total CARBONS NET 4.42 g, Cal 344 , Fat 30.38 g, Carbs 10.03 g, Fiber 5.61 g, Protein 8.26 g

CROCKPOT STRAWBERRY DUMP CAKE

Ingredients

- 15.25 oz Betty Crocker Strawberry Cake Mix {1 box}
- 42 oz Strawberry pie filling {2 boxes of 21 oz Each}
- ½ cup melted butter

Instructions

4. Spray nonstick cooking spray into the Crockpot.

5. Strawberry pie Fill the empty boxes at the bottom of the Crockpot and distribute them evenly.

6. Mix the dry cake mix with melted butter in a medium bowl and stir until it crumbles. Break large pieces into small pieces of spoon}.

7. Pour the cake / crumbled butter mixture into the Crockpot over the strawberries and distribute it evenly over the jar with a lid.

8. Cook 2 hours HIGH or 4 hours DOWN.

9. Use ice or whipped cream for drinking. ALWAYS !!

Prep time: 5 min; **Servings:** 8

Macros: Total CARBONS NET 4.42 g, Cal 344 , Fat 30.38 g, Carbs 10.03 g, Fiber 5.61 g, Protein 8.26 g

RED VELVET PIE

Ingredients

- ½ cup apple sauce

- 1 cup water

- 3 eggs

- 15.25 oz Duncan Hines Red Velvet Cake Mix {1 can}

Instructions

5. Mix all the ingredients with a blender for 1 minute.

6. Spray cooking spray in crockpot.

7. Pour and cover the mixture in the crockpot.

8. Bake for 1.5 to 2 hours or until cooked over medium heat.

9. Once the cake is made, I just carefully cut the pieces of Crockpot.

10. Also, enjoy the addition of some of your favorite glazes!

11. Serve with ENJOY and ice cream !!

Prep time: 15 min; Servings: 12

Macros: 380 Cal, 17 g total fat, 5 g saturated fat, 54 g total Carbs

LEMON MOUSSE WITH LIME CREAM AND ROASTED NUTS

Ingredients

- ¼ cup chopped English walnuts

- 9 Tbsp fresh lemon juice

- 3 large eggs (whole)

- 3 large egg yolks

- 6 packs of Stevia

- 2 Tbsp unsalted butter bar

- 3/4 cup heavy cream

- 5 Tbsp fresh lime juice

Instructions

1. Use a zester, the thin side of a box grater, or a micro plane to grate lemons and limes.

2. Preheat the oven to 400° F. Place the nuts on a baking sheet and bake until golden brown, about 8 min, taking care not to burn.

3. Boil a large pot of water or a double boiler.

4. Lemon zest and juice. Put the taste and the liquid in a medium bowl or on a double kettle. Add whole eggs and yolks. Put the pan on the boiling water and reduce heat. Beat the eggs, yolks, and lemon juice with a hand mixer until the mixture is creamy and the volume doubles. Keep away from heat. Put the butter and 4 packets of sugar substitute in the bowl and let the mixture cool.

5. Put the cream in a mixing bowl. Peel and squeeze the files, as shown above. Add to the cream. Beat the lime and cream mixture until soft peaks appear. Add 2 packs of stevia.

6. Place the first half of the lime cream in 4 glasses of parfait or martini, then a third of the nuts, followed by the whole lemon curd. Then add another layer of nuts and cover them with the rest of the lime cream.

Prep time: 15 min; **Servings:** 4

Macros: 6.9 g net Carbs 9 g protein 34.2 g fat 1.5 g fiber 362.3 Cal

ALMOND PANNA COTTA

Ingredients

- 1 cup heavy cream

- 1 cup unsweetened vanilla milk with almond breeze

- 2 packages of sucralose sweetener

- 2 tsp pure almond extract

- 1 ½ tsp powdered gelatin (sugar-free)

Instructions

1. This dessert must be cooled for at least 4 hours.

2. Pour ½ cup heavy cream into a bowl. Sprinkle with jelly and let stand until soft.

3. Mix the remaining heavy cream with the almond milk in a small saucepan. Heat over medium heat until tiny bubbles begin to form along the sides of the pan.

4. For the gelatin mixture, add the sugar substitute and stir to mix well.

5. Once the mixture is cold, add the almond extract. For ⅓ cup mixture into each of the 6 plastic cups or decorative shapes. Cover with plastic wrap and let cool overnight or until ready, at least 4 hours.

6. Put each panna cotta on a plate to serve. Garnish with optional sliced almonds.

Prep time: 20 min; **Servings:** 6

Macros: 1.4 g net Carbs 1.5 g protein 15.1 g fat 0.2 g fiber 151.6 Cal

ALMOND WITH CHOCOLATE SAUCE AND CHERRY GARNISH

Ingredients

3. 1 cup sliced almonds

4. 1 tsp of baking powder (straight phosphate, double effect)

5. A pinch of of tartar

6. 5 large eggs (whole)

7. ½ cup sucralose sweetener (sugar substitute)

8. 2 portions of sugar-free chocolate bar

9. 2 g of baked chocolate, sugar-free

10. 16 tsp sugar syrup and hazelnuts

11. 6 Tbsp heavy cream

12. 1 our liquid tap water

13. 1 ½ cups frozen cherries

14. 1 serving of low-carb wheat bread

Instructions

4. Use the to make low-carb wheat bread for this . You need a slice. You will also need ⅓ cup unsweetened hazelnut syrup.

5. Heat the oven to 350° F.

6. Spread almonds on a baking sheet and roast until golden, about 10 min, totally cool. If your bread is not old, toast the dough with the almonds. Transfer to food processor and add the bread, baking powder, and cream of tartar; mix until almonds are finely ground.

7. Line a 9-inch spring font with waxed paper. Lightly spray with an oil spray and sprinkle with about 1 tsp ground almonds.

8. Combine 5 egg yolks and ¼ cup crystalline sugar substitute in a large bowl; beat with an electric mixer until soft and fluffy, about 3 min Beat 5 Protein in another bowl with clean, dry whisks until soft peaks occur. Add ¼ cup the remaining sugar substitute (keep 1 tsp for the whipped cream filling) and beat until stiff peaks form about 3 min

9. Fold the walnuts in yellow in 3 additions, interspersed each time with a quarter of the Protein; fold in the remaining goals. Spread in the pan. Bake until a toothpick in the middle comes out clean, 18 to 20 min

10. Let cool in a pan on a wire rack. Release a sharp knife between the cake and the container. Remove the waxed paper and turn it over on a serving platter.

11. Mix the chocolate, hazelnut syrup, and 2 Tbsp cream on a double boiler with boiling water. Beat until the chocolate melts, then stir in 2 Tbsp water. In a bowl, beat 4 Tbsp cream into soft wedges with ½ tsp crystalline sugar substitute.

12. Cut the cake into 8 pieces; Cover with sauce. Place the whipped cream next to the cake and add the thawed cherries.

Prep time: 25 min; **Servings:** 8

Macros: 7.5 g net Carbs 9.9 g protein 19.9 g fat 4 g fiber 250.8 Cal Cal

CUISINE BROWNIES

Ingredients

5. 4 oz squares of baking chocolate without sugar

6. ½ cup unsalted butter bar

7. ½ cup heavy cream

8. 5 large eggs (whole)

9. 1 cup sucralose sweetener

10. 2 tsp of baking powder (straight phosphate, double effect)

11. 4 ½ Servings:, flour mixture

Instructions

1. Use the to make the flour mixture for this . You should have 1 ¼ cups of the flour mixture.

2. Preheat the oven to 325 ° F.

3. Place the unsweetened chocolate and butter in a robust bowl and microwave for about 2 min until the chocolate melts. Beat in heavy cream.

4. In another bowl, add the eggs and 1 cup crystalline sugar substitute. Beat with an electric mixer until the mixture is homogeneous. Reduce the blender on low speed and mix the chocolate mixture.

5. Combine baking powder and 1 ¼ cups low-carb baking mixture with a wooden spoon.

6. Cover the 8 x 8-inch pan with a spray of non-stick vegetable oil and distribute the mixture evenly in the pan.

7. Bake 30 to 35 min at 325 ° F or until cooked through (stick in the middle comes out clean). (Do not overcook, otherwise, the brownies will become dry and hard).

8. Once cool, cut into 5 rows for 5 rows to make 25 brownies.

Prep time: 15 min; **Pieces:** 25

Macros: 2.7 g net Carbs 5.5 g protein 9.4 g fat 1.2 g fiber 114.7 Cal Cal

CAKE CRUST

Ingredients

- ⅓ cup stone-ground 100% whole grain puff pastry flour

- ⅓ cup whole wheat flour

- 2 g of vital wheat gluten

- 3 Tbsp soft wheat germ

- ½ tsp salt

- ½ cup unsalted butter bar

- 1 Tbsp tap water

Instructions

1. In a food processor, mix flour, wheat gluten, germ, salt, and butter until mixture looks like a full meal. Slowly add water and continue pressing until the dough begins to merge. Flip a sheet of plastic, form a balefully, and cover with plastic. Flatten on a 7-inch disc and let cool in the freezer for 15 min

2. Roll out the dough between 2 sheets of plastic wrap in a 12-inch circle (if necessary, sprinkle ½ tsp wheat gluten flour on each side for easier rolling). Remove the top plastic sheet and turn it into a 9-inch cake pan. Center the dough and press on the bottom and sides of the plate. Remove the plastic, roll under the edges and shrink decorative. Put in the freezer for 15 min

3. Use the raw crust as directed in the of your choice. Or preheat the oven on a pre-baked coat at 400° F. Pierce the bottom and corners of the mold with a fork. Cover the lid of the cake with aluminum foil, fill it halfway with cake weights or dried beans and turn the paper to cover the edge of the dough. Bake for 16 min Remove aluminum foil and weights, lightly cover with aluminum foil and bake for 4 to 6 minutes more or until golden. Let it cool on a rack for 20 min.

Prep time: 10 min; **Servings:** 8

Macros: 3.6 g net Carbs 8.6 g protein 13.2 g fat 1.3 g fiber 168.2 Cal Cal

CONCLUSION